SMART
Wellness Workbook

Cultural wisdom meets modern brain science

Reba Peoples, M.D.

S.M.A.R.T. WELLNESS® WORKBOOK

S.M.A.R.T. WELLNESS is a trademark of Imara Health and Wellness, PLLC

Balboa Press books may be ordered through booksellers or by contacting:

Balboa Press
A Division of Hay House
1663 Liberty Drive
Bloomington, IN 47403
www.balboapress.com
1 (877) 407-4847

Because of the dynamic nature of the Internet, any web addresses or links contained in this book may have changed since publication and may no longer be valid. The views expressed in this work are solely those of the author and do not necessarily reflect the views of the publisher, and the publisher hereby disclaims any responsibility for them.

Any people depicted in stock imagery provided by Getty Images are models, and such images are being used for illustrative purposes only.
Certain stock imagery © Getty Images.

ISBN: 978-1-9822-1907-9 (sc)
ISBN: 978-1-9822-1906-2 (e)

Print information available on the last page.

Balboa Press rev. date: 01/22/2019

BALBOA.
PRESS
A DIVISION OF HAY HOUSE

Congratulations on making the SMART decision to invest in your own wellness!

As a holistic psychiatrist, founder of Imara Health and Wellness and creator of SMART Wellness®, I often work with people just like yourself who would love to feel energized, enthusiastic and motivated in their day-to-day lives but often find themselves struggling with feelings of burnout, frustration or overwhelm. With so much on the to-do list, finding time for wellness can often feel like an impossible task.

Like yourself, I've also battled feelings of overwhelm and struggled with making the commitment to prioritize my own health. The SMART Wellness® method is the direct result of many years of lessons learned from both professional study and personal application.

Although it hasn't always been easy, making the commitment to incorporate SMART Wellness® choices into my daily life has allowed me to make the shift from feeling stressed out, overwhelmed and defeated to confident, capable and in control.

Today, I can confidently say that my life is one of joy, clarity, and purpose. My mission is to help you learn SMART ways to harness both the power of ancient wisdom and the gift of modern brain science in order to build an extraordinary life that is healthy, joyful and purpose-driven.

The tools outlined in this workbook will distill the SMART Wellness® principles into an easy, uncomplicated roadmap that will help you incorporate wellness principles into your daily life right away. I'm so excited to partner with you on your healing journey.

Let's get started!

Dr. Reba
PEOPLES

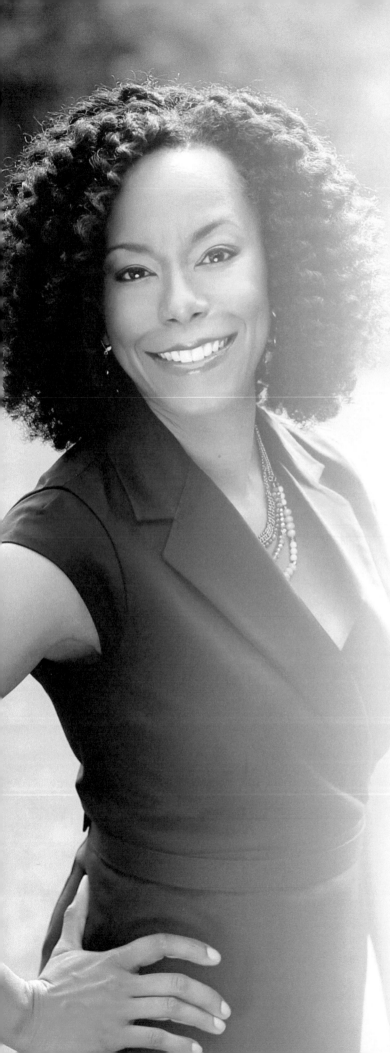

SLEEP

Your secret weapon for regulating stress hormones, cultivating brain health and improving physical vitality. Learning good sleep hygiene practices can help you get the restful, restorative sleep that your body needs.

MOVEMENT

Getting active is a major tool for getting healthy– not only physically, but emotionally as well. Incorporating regular physical activity into your daily routine can help boost your mood and reduce your risk of chronic disease.

AWARENESS

One can think of awareness as the ability to recognize our thoughts, feelings, sensations, and environment as they truly are. Mindful awareness allows us to experience these aspects of consciousness without judgment or attachment.

RECOGNITION OF IDENTITY

Knowing who you are is one of the first steps in building a purpose-driven life that is in alignment with your values. Your personal history, family history, and cultural history play key roles in shaping your understanding of yourself and the world around you.

TAILOR YOUR INPUTS

It is important to carefully choose how you feed your body, mind, and spirit. Although most of us recognize the importance of caring for our physical bodies via proper nutrition and avoiding environmental toxins, we must also be mindful of how we feed our minds and nurture our spirits.

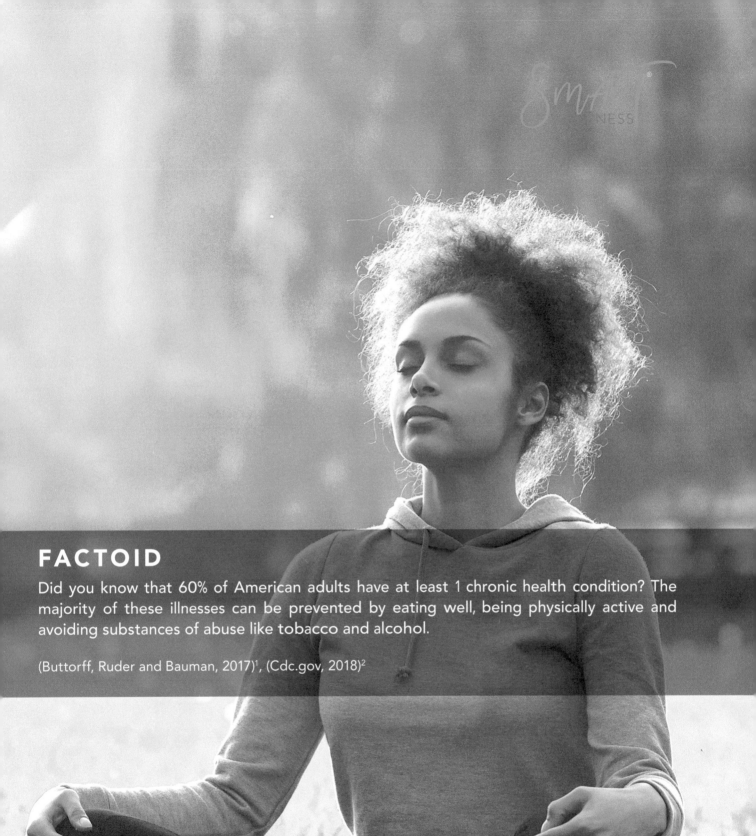

FACTOID

Did you know that 60% of American adults have at least 1 chronic health condition? The majority of these illnesses can be prevented by eating well, being physically active and avoiding substances of abuse like tobacco and alcohol.

(Buttorff, Ruder and Bauman, 2017)[1], (Cdc.gov, 2018)[2]

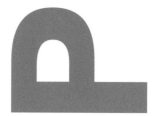
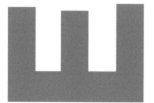
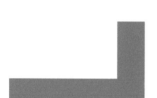
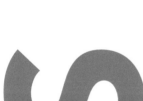
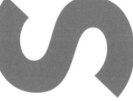

Proper sleep hygiene is key in getting restful, restorative sleep.

Develop a routine
- Commit to 7-9 hours of sleep nightly.
- Incorporate a mindfulness practice such as tai chi, chi gong or stretching to quiet your mind before bedtime.
- Consider an evening ritual such as a foot soak, bath or aromatherapy.

Create healthy habits
- Use your bed only for sleeping – resist the urge to read or watch television in bed.
- Eat multiple small meals throughout the day to avoid blood sugar dips at night.
- Avoid strenuous exercise less than three hours before bedtime.
- Avoid stimulants such as caffeine during evening hours.
- Avoid alcohol as a sleep aid. Although drinking alcohol may cause you to feel 'sleepy', alcohol intake actually prevents you from reaching the deeper, restorative phases of sleep.
- Avoid long-term use of sleep-promoting hormones like melatonin unless directed to do so by your medical provider. Generally, melatonin should only be used short-term for a maximum of 2 weeks.

Cultivate a restful environment
- Make sure that your bedroom or sleeping area is free of artificial light sources. Consider investing in an eye mask or blackout curtains.
- Make to maintain your bedroom at a cool and comfortable temperature for sleeping.

Be mindful of blue light exposure
- Blue light suppresses production of melatonin - our body's natural sleep hormone.
- Use a blue light filter (night mode on most devices) or blue light blocking glasses when using electronic devices after dark.

Be mindful of electromagnetic radiation
- Although this area remains somewhat controversial, there is early evidence that Wi-Fi,
- 4G, Bluetooth and other EMR sources have the potential to disrupt sleep architecture and make it difficult to obtain a restful night's sleep.
- Be sure to power off your devices before bed.
- Remove Wi-Fi routers from the bedroom.
- Sleep with cell phones as far away from your body as possible if unable to power down or switch to airplane mode at night.

How many hours of sleep are you getting each night?

Do you feel rested in the morning?

What are some action steps that you can take to improve the quality of your sleep?

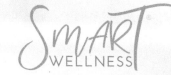

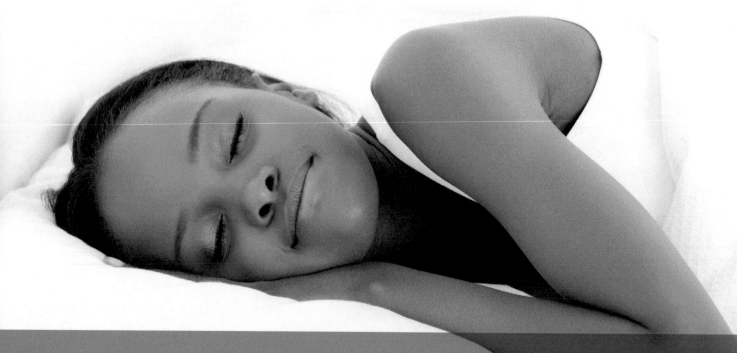

FACTOID

Did you know that 7-9 hours is the ideal amount of time to sleep nightly? Individuals who sleep less than 6 hours nightly or more than 10 hours nightly are significantly more likely to struggle with obesity, frequent mental distress, heart disease, stroke, and diabetes.

(Liu et al., 2013)[3]

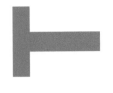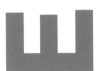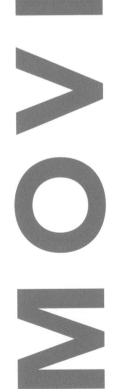

MOVEMENT

Did you know that regular physical activity helps regulate stress hormones?

We don't have to become elite athletes or join the local CrossFit to reap the benefits of moving our bodies. Even simple activities like walking or stretching can have a big impact on our physical and emotional health. Here are some fun and simple ways to bring more movement into your life.

Get Moving
- Take the stairs instead of the elevator if going up or down only 1-2 flights of stairs.
- Stand for 30 seconds after every 20 minutes of seated activity.
- Replace in-office meetings with walking meetings.
- Commit to 10 minutes of gentle stretching each morning.
- Invest in a pedometer and make it a goal to log 10,000 steps daily.

Get FITT
Once you're ready to graduate into more vigorous exercise, it is important to be clear about the Frequency, Intensity, Time and Type of exercise that you plan to incorporate.

Frequency: How often do you plan to do your identified activity?

Intensity: How much effort or intensity will you extend?

Time: How long will you spend on the activity?

Type: What will you do?

The more specific your goal, the more likely you are to achieve it. Rather than stating that you plan to work out more, a more specific FITT goal would be to state that you plan to run on the treadmill (Type), for 30 minutes (Time) at 4mph (Intensity) after work every Monday, Wednesday and Friday (Frequency)

How many hours per day would you estimate that you spend sitting down?

Are you happy with your current amount of daily physical activity?

If not, what is a realistic goal for incorporating more movement into your life?

Remember to use the FITT acronym as a guide to help you think about what type of activity you plan to incorporate, how often would you like to do it, how much effort you plan to exert and how much time you will devote to your chosen activity:

Frequency:_____

Intensity:_____

Time:_____

Type:_____

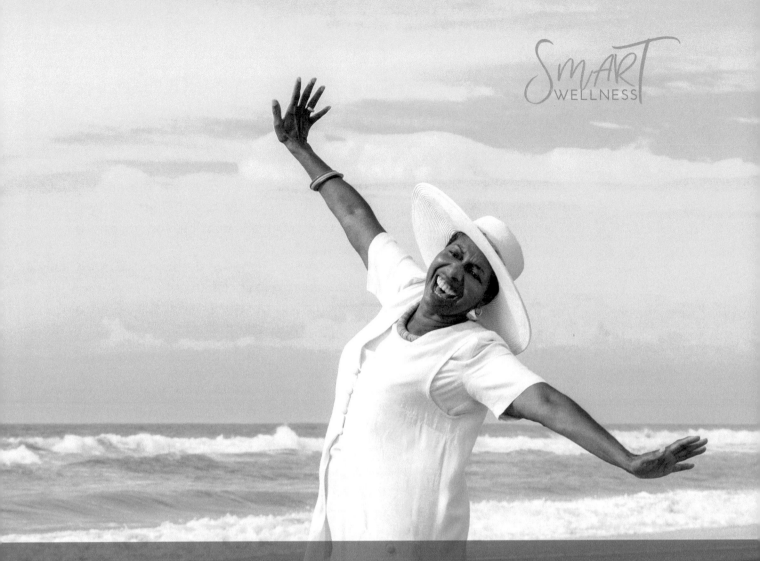

FACTOID

Did you know that our prehistoric ancestors walked an average of 14,960 steps per day while modern Amish communities walk an average of 16,310 steps per day? This is in contrast to most modern Americans who walk an average of only 5,126 steps daily. This historically unprecedented amount of physical inactivity is one of the primary drivers of our modern chronic disease epidemic. If we want to ensure that we get healthy, we have to ensure that we get moving!

(Booth, Roberts and Laye, 2012)[4]

AWARENESS

Did you know that the average American is estimated to have an average of 50,000 thoughts in a single day?

For most of us, the majority of those thoughts (~65%) are negative. Those automatic negative thoughts, or ANTS for short, can have a devastating impact on how we view ourselves and what we believe is possible for our future.

Individuals with a tendency toward automatic negative thoughts are more likely to struggle with symptoms of depression and social anxiety. These thoughts stop us from pursuing our goals and rob us of reaching our full potential due to the immobilizing fear caused by worrying about all of the ways that things could possibly go wrong.

Mindful awareness not only allows us to become aware of our thoughts, feelings, sensations, and environment, it also enables us to learn to experience them without judgment or attachment. According to neuroscientist Jill Bolte Taylor, our emotions are chemically active in our brains for a mere 90 seconds. Beyond this initial 90 seconds, it is up to us to consciously decide if we will allow the emotion (be it positive or negative) to persist. If we allow whatever negative emotion that we may be experiencing in a given moment to run its course without judgment and without resistance, we will be able to allow the unwanted emotion to dissipate and exit our physical and emotional awareness naturally. Given this quirk in our physiology, resisting the unwanted emotion is ironically what allows it to persist. Being brave enough to allow yourself to experience it without judgment is what will allow it to pass.

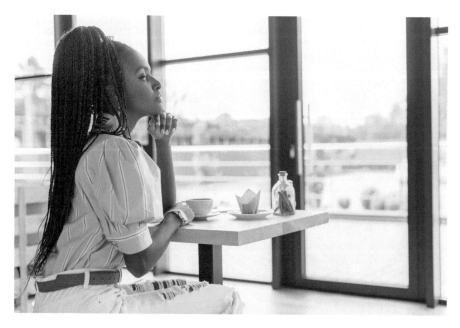

Do you feel that you are able to devote enough time to reflection, planning and creative thinking?

If so, what big dreams are you currently pursuing?

If not, what barriers are standing in the way of having more time to devote to rest and personal reflection?

What are some ways that you can overcome those barriers?

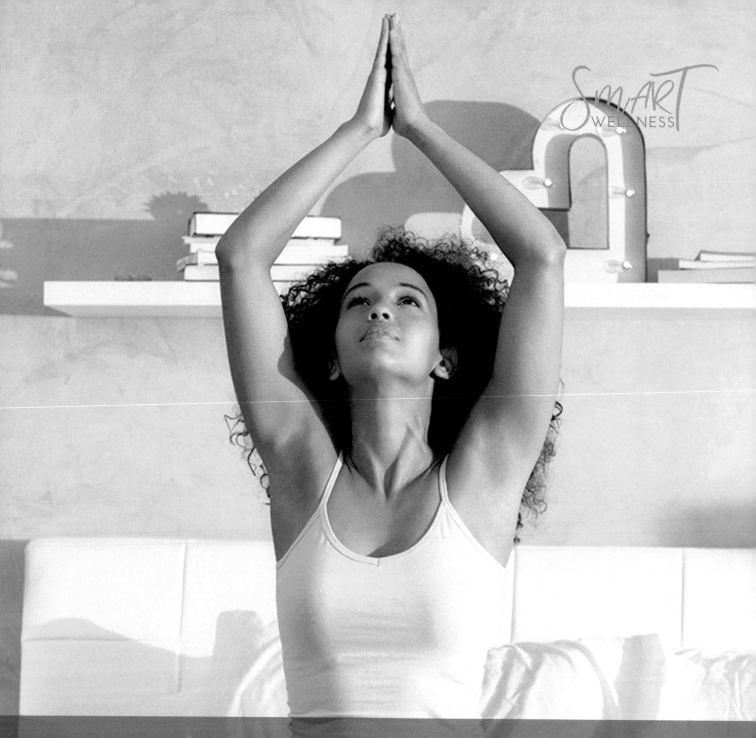

FACTOID

Did you know that having a regular mindfulness practice can actually change the structure of your brain? People who engage in a regular mindfulness practice have changes in the areas of the brain that are associated with sustaining attention and regulating emotions.

(Hölzel et al., 2011)[5]

RECOGNITION IDENTITY

Knowing who you are is one of the first steps in building a purpose-driven life that is in alignment with your values.

We all have a history – not only a personal history but a family history and a cultural history as well. Each of these histories play a key role in shaping our understanding of ourselves and the world around us.

Your personal history has to do with all of the individual experiences that have led up to this point in your life. The circumstances of your birth, the people who raised you, the place where you grew up, and major life events - both triumphs and challenges - have an important influence on how you see yourself and how you navigate the world.

Your family history has to do with the collective experiences of your immediate and extended family members. Whether your family is biological or chosen, family is one of the earliest and most influential models that we have in learning how to relate to others. Often times, our current relationships are reflective of relationship patterns that we have seen modeled by family members while growing up. If we are not aware of those patterns –both positive and not so positive – we may repeat dysfunctional relationship patterns in our current relationships without even being aware that we are doing so. Once we become aware of these patterns, we are able to make better choices and model how we would like to be treated by others.

Your cultural history has to do with the collective, historical experiences of your ancestors and the present-day cultural and social factors that have been shaped by history. According to Dr. Wade Nobles, culture gives us a general design for living and patterns for interpreting our reality. It is important to understand culture and history because not understanding our history can cause a major blind spot in our understanding of self.

What personal values have been most important in shaping your life?

What family values have been the most important in shaping your life?

What cultural values have been most important in shaping your life?

Do you feel that you are currently living a life that is in alignment with your values?

Why or why not?

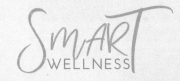

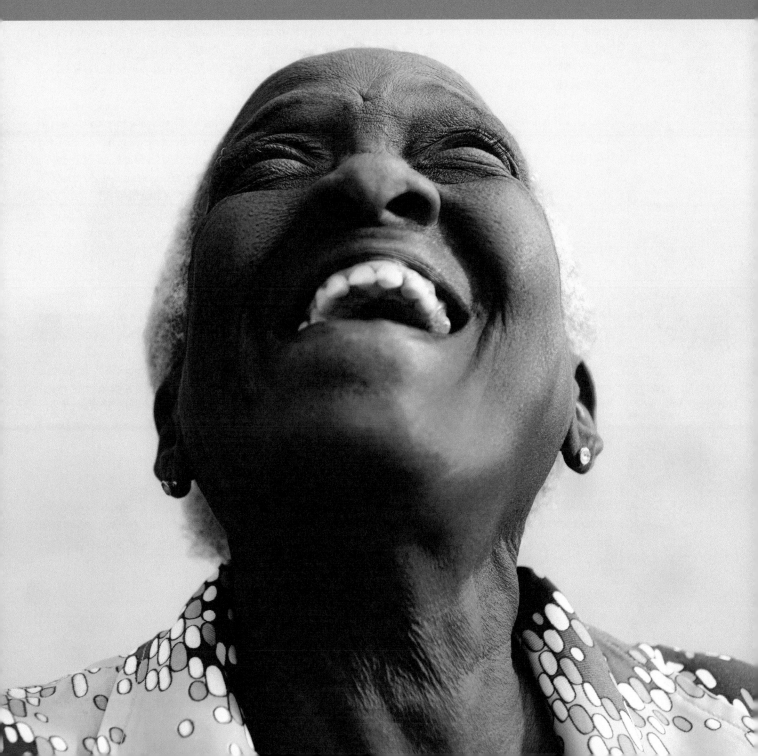

FACTOID

Did you know that self-awareness is an important precursor to self- compassion? Being kind to yourself isn't just an airy fairy notion. Clinical research has shown that self-compassion can be a powerful tool for improving mood and combating negative emotions.

(Odou and Brinker, 2013)[6]

TAILOR YOUR INPUTS

Are you as careful about what you choose to feed your mind and spirit as you are about what you choose to feed your physical body?

Although most of us recognize the importance of caring for our physical bodies via proper nutrition and avoiding environmental toxins, we must also be mindful of how we feed our minds and nurture our spirits.

Body

One of the best protections that we have against the ravaging effects of daily exposure to toxic stress is fueling our bodies A variety of colorful, nutritious whole foods. A general rule of thumb is that if something comes in a bag, a box, or a can it probably should not go into your body. Make an effort to commit to avoiding processed foods and refined sugars. Your brain and body will thank you.

Although many of us are very aware of the critical role that the food that we eat can have on the way that we feel, many of us do not know that what we put on our body is just as important as what we put into it. Did you know that the average American exposes his or her body to hundreds of synthetic chemicals every day? This is a problem because an estimated 20 to 60% of the chemicals that we put onto our skin are directly absorbed into our bodies. Many of the chemicals that are commonly used as additives in our makeup, personal care products, and household cleaners have the potential to act as toxins in our brains, cause cancers or act as endocrine disruptors that can dysregulate our hormones.

Mind

Don't overlook the influence of media on your emotional health. Marketers have an incentive to exploit our insecurities and profit from our fears. Repeatedly exposing our minds to messages and images that trigger the stress response can have a profoundly negative impact on our physical and emotional health. Excessive consumption of media is associated with lowered creativity and a lower capacity for reflection, critical thinking, and analysis. Make a commitment to set aside time each day to read or listen to something positive or educational. Some of the most successful people in the world adhere to the five-hour-rule. This means that they spend an average of one hour each weekday engaged in learning something new.

Soul

Toxic relationships can also be an overlooked source of stress. Are you spending the majority of your time with people who are positive and supportive or with people who are negative and emotionally draining? If you feel worse about yourself after spending time with someone you may want to reevaluate the relationship.

Spirit

Viktor Frankl once wrote that the meaning of life is to give life meaning. Life is an amazing and precious gift. It is up to each of us to find a purpose that feeds our spirit and allows our soul to evolve.

ACTION PLAN

BODY

1. Stay hydrated! A general rule of thumb is to drink 0.5-1 ounce of water per pound of body weight daily. For example, a 150-pound individual should aim to drink ~75-150 ounces of water daily. Given your current body weight, what is your daily water intake goal?
   - Body weight in pounds =_____
   - Minimum daily water intake in ounces =_____(divide your weight in pounds by 2)
   - Ideal daily water intake in ounces =_____(your weight in pounds)

2. Eat real food. Try to avoid processed foods and refined sugars during your next trip to the grocery store. Remember to read labels. If there are any chemical additives or preservatives on the label, think twice about purchasing.

3. Create a healthy environment. Take an inventory of your current cosmetics and household cleaners by using the tools at ewg.org

The skin-deep cosmetics database will allow you to identify the safety of the ingredients contained in your cosmetics. You can even customize a reading by typing in the individual ingredients on the label if your particular brand of cosmetic is not listed in the database (https://www.ewg.org/skindeep).

EWG's healthy living guide will help you identify the safety of the chemicals found in household products such as cleaners, air fresheners, paint, furniture, and carpeting (https://www.ewg. org/healthyhomeguide).

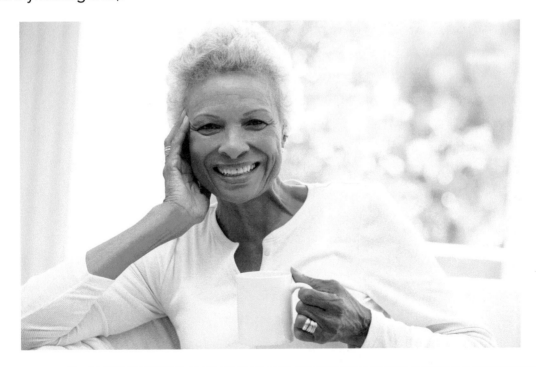

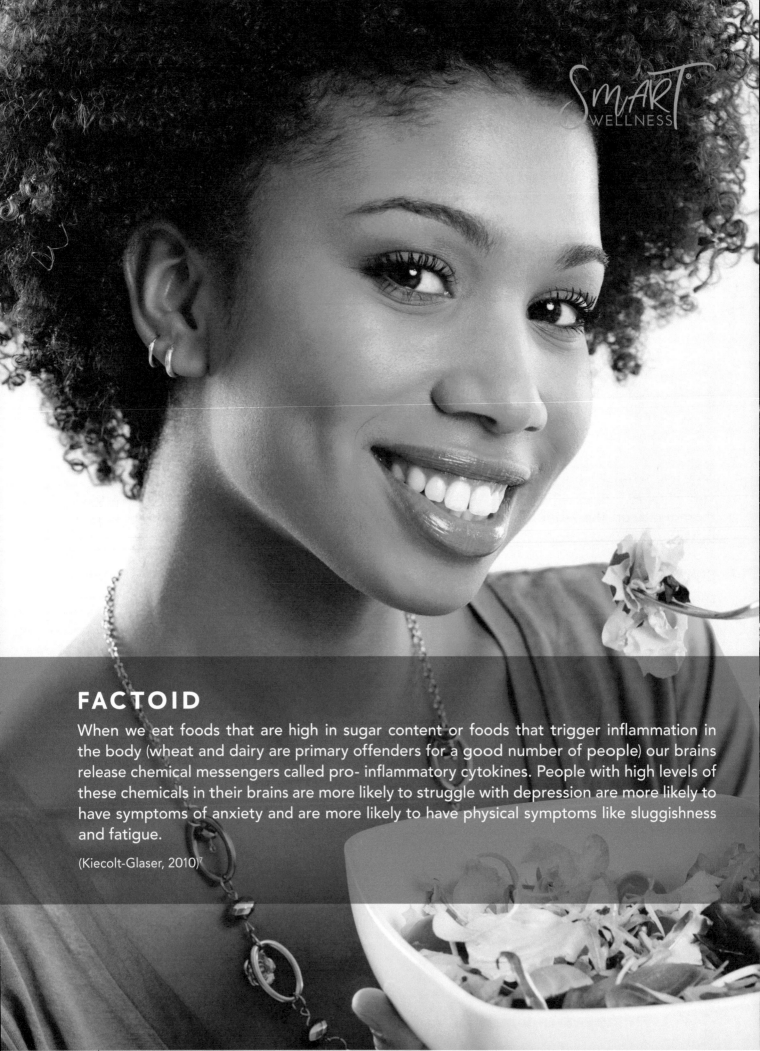

FACTOID

When we eat foods that are high in sugar content or foods that trigger inflammation in the body (wheat and dairy are primary offenders for a good number of people) our brains release chemical messengers called pro- inflammatory cytokines. People with high levels of these chemicals in their brains are more likely to struggle with depression are more likely to have symptoms of anxiety and are more likely to have physical symptoms like sluggishness and fatigue.

(Kiecolt-Glaser, 2010)[7]

ACTION PLAN

MIND

On an average day, how much time do you estimate that you spend watching television or consuming social media?

When is the last time that you read or listened to something inspiring or educational outside of work or school assignments?

What is one thing that you can do to feed your mind positive or inspiring information?

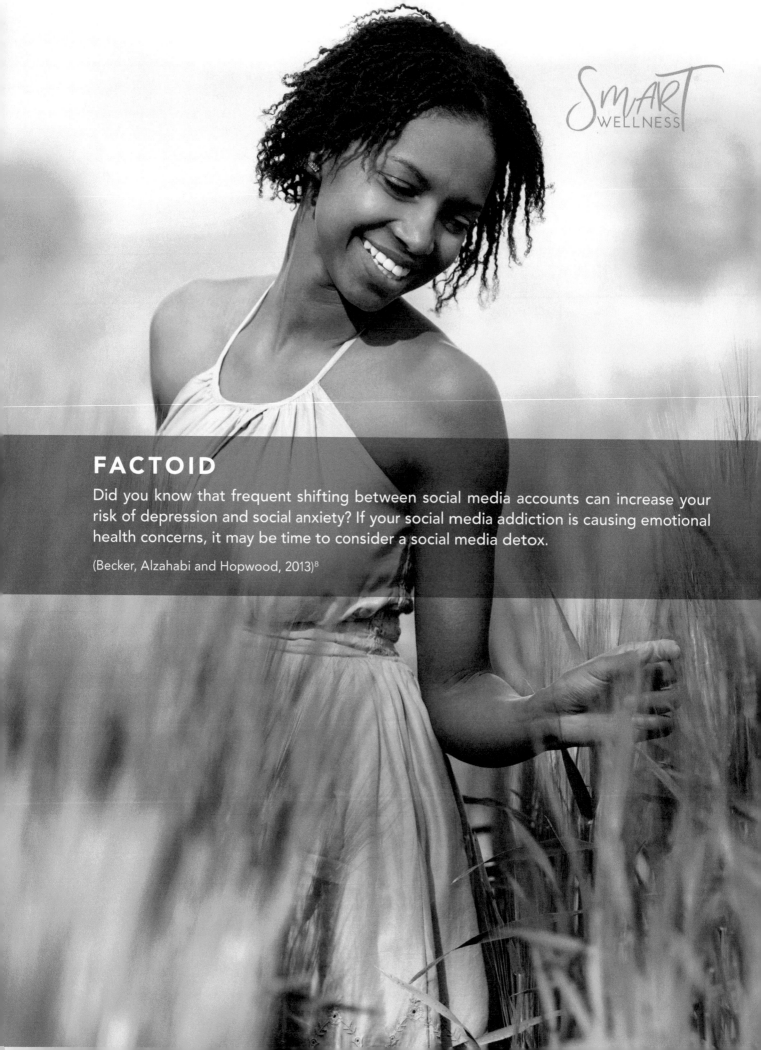

FACTOID

Did you know that frequent shifting between social media accounts can increase your risk of depression and social anxiety? If your social media addiction is causing emotional health concerns, it may be time to consider a social media detox.

(Becker, Alzahabi and Hopwood, 2013)[8]

ACTION PLAN

SOUL AND SPIR IT

When is the last time that you reached out to a friend or an acquaintance to spend time together socially?

What are you most passionate about?

What are your biggest strengths and spiritual gifts?

How are you using those gifts to bring you closer to your purpose?

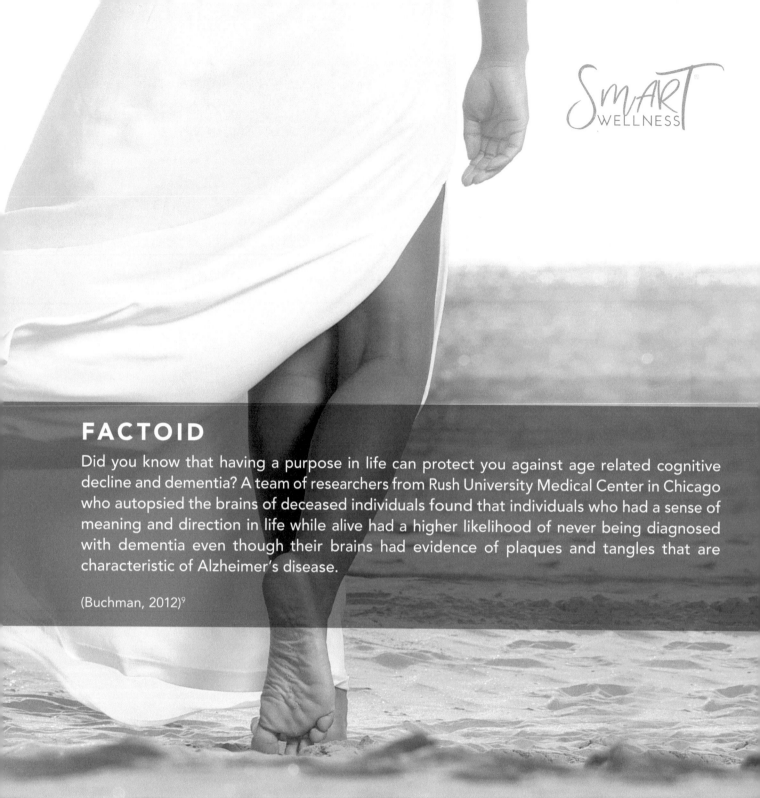

WELLNESS

FACTOID

Did you know that having a purpose in life can protect you against age related cognitive decline and dementia? A team of researchers from Rush University Medical Center in Chicago who autopsied the brains of deceased individuals found that individuals who had a sense of meaning and direction in life while alive had a higher likelihood of never being diagnosed with dementia even though their brains had evidence of plaques and tangles that are characteristic of Alzheimer's disease.

(Buchman, 2012)[9]

NOTES

Endnotes

1. Buttorff, C., Ruder, T. and Bauman, M. (2017). Multiple Chronic Conditions in the United States. [online] Santa Monica, California: RAND Corporation. Available at: http://ISBN: 978-0-8330-9737-8 [Accessed 16 Sep. 2018].

2. Cdc.gov. (2018). About Chronic Disease | Chronic Disease Prevention and Health Promotion | CDC. [online] Available at: https://www.cdc.gov/chronicdisease/about/index.htm [Accessed 23 Sep. 2018].

3. Liu, Y., Wheaton, A., Chapman, D. and Croft, J. (2013). Sleep Duration and Chronic Diseases among US Adults Age 45 Years and Older: Evidence From the 2010 Behavioral Risk Factor Surveillance System. Sleep, 36(10), pp.1421-1427.

4. Booth, F., Roberts, C. and Laye, M. (2012). Lack of Exercise Is a Major Cause of Chronic Diseases. Comprehensive Physiology.

5. Hölzel, B., Carmody, J., Vangel, M., Congleton, C., Yerramsetti, S., Gard, T. and Lazar, S. (2011). Mindfulness practice leads to increases in regional brain gray matter density. Psychiatry Research: Neuroimaging, 191(1), pp.36-43.

6. Odou, N. and Brinker, J. (2013). Exploring the Relationship between Rumination, Self-compassion, and Mood. Self and Identity, 13(4), pp.449-459.

7. Kiecolt-Glaser, J. (2010). Stress, Food, and Inflammation: Psychoneuroimmunology and Nutrition at the Cutting Edge. Psychosomatic Medicine, 72(4), pp.365-369.

8. Becker, M., Alzahabi, R. and Hopwood, C. (2013). Media Multitasking Is Associated with Symptoms of Depression and Social Anxiety. Cyberpsychology, Behavior, and Social Networking, 16(2), pp.132-135.

9. Buchman, A. (2012). Effect of Purpose in Life on the Relation Between Alzheimer Disease Pathologic Changes on Cognitive Function in Advanced Age. Archives of General Psychiatry, 69(5), p.499.

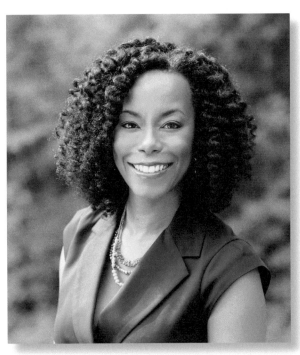

Congratulations on completing the workbook!

You've learned some great strategies for building a wellness practice that will allow you to optimize your physical, emotional and spiritual health. If you would like to learn more great strategies for incorporating wellness into your daily life, be sure to visit www. imarahealthandwellness.com

Be well and God bless,

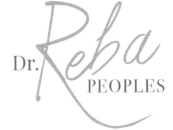

Dr. Reba PEOPLES

Printed in the United States
By Bookmasters